Living Better while Living with Pain

21 Ways to Reduce the Stress of Chronic Pain and Create Greater Ease and Relief TODAY

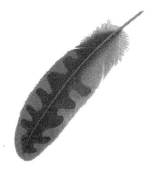

SARAH ANNE SHOCKLEY

Any Road Press

Fairfax, California

for all my relations

CONTENTS

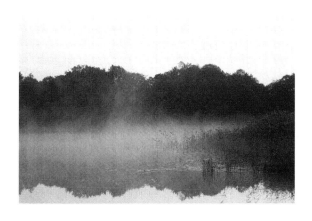

1
WHY THIS BOOK

IF YOU ARE living with pain, day in and day out, then we have something in common. Like you, I have had my life altered dramatically by the presence of chronic physical pain.

My pain arrived with a work-related injury and never left because the condition has not healed, even after 8 years. Every part of my life - my ability to work, my relationships, what I can and can't do for pleasure, and all the mundane tasks of daily life - have been hugely impacted.

In a deposition for Workmen's Compensation, my employer's lawyer asked me, "What in your life has been affected by this injury?" I looked at her, wondering if she had even the vaguest clue about my condition. Where to even begin?

My body burned and ached intensely from head to foot, I could barely use my hands for anything practical, my neck wouldn't turn, I seldom slept more than a few hours a night and never more than about 40 minutes at a time, I had PTSD, and my brain was on fire.

"Everything," I said.

"Everything?" she asked, sounding incredulous.

"Everything," I said, with emphasis. Then I left the room abruptly so I wouldn't have to cry in front of her.

LIVING IN CONSTANT, often acute, pain has been one of the most challenging things I have ever had to endure in my life. If you are in pain now, you know what I mean. Chronic pain is relentless, unforgiving, torturous, exhausting, and mostly invisible to others.

During my time with pain, I have often felt very alone. In the beginning, I didn't know anyone who was going through anything similar to me, and I didn't feel well enough or have the energy to seek out or attend a support group, if there even was one. I needed something close at hand, like this book, to act as a companion through the pain.

But I never discovered one.

Most of the books I did find on chronic pain were written by doctors and other medical practitioners and they focused mostly on physical remedies and manipulations. They undoubtedly had their benefits for many people, but they didn't offer me what I needed in terms of emotional support, solace, and practical everyday advice.

Personally, I didn't so much need to hear from someone who was a specialist in pain, I needed to hear from someone who had lived with deep pain day in and day out for an extended period of time.

I needed to hear from someone like me.

This is why I'm writing this book now, to offer you a few bits of practical advice that I wish I'd known at the beginning of my journey. I hope they will help you get through the very difficult challenges of living with chronic pain - pain that others most often can't see or understand - with a bit more ease and well-being.

The ideas I present here are suggestions for what to do beyond using pain medications. I am not opposed to pain medications, since they can be incredibly useful. But sometimes, as has been the case with me, they simply don't work, or they may come with nasty side effects. And, there is the very real concern of using them over the long term in terms of possible addiction and negative effects on the overall health of the body.

So the ideas presented here do not rely on pain medication, nor do they require you to stop using them either. They are suggestions for working with pain and lessening pain that you can initiate and maintain yourself, with the overall goal of not *killing* pain, per se, but working with it and through it to come to a place of true healing.

This is a concise guide, so we will get right to the heart of the matter. For further information, free resources, additional books and The Pain Companion Blog, I invite you to visit me at my website: www.thepaincompanion.com.

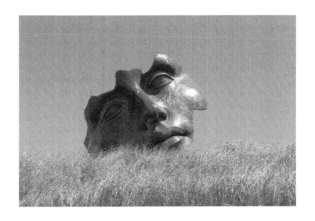

2
WHY AM I STILL HURTING?

WE EXPECT ALL pain to be short-lived, so being in pain over many weeks, months and even years, often leads to confusion and frustration. What is going on?

It may seem almost like a sign of failure when you can't stop the pain you are in. Your body is not responding positively to the therapies and approaches of a medical system in which very many highly intelligent people believe. It isn't working for you, and in some ways, this can feel like your fault.

You may feel like you should work harder, or hide your pain, or downplay it so you don't have to keep reporting that nothing is working.

You may feel really bad about the fact that you, of all people in the world, aren't responding to the medical options presented to you.

You may feel frustrated with yourself, thinking that you should have been able to end the pain by now, to have healed the condition, and to be done with this so you can move on.

Or you may feel angry, disappointed or frustrated with the shortcomings of the medical world. It seems that somehow something isn't being done in the right way. It's very difficult to come to the conclusion that the help you need just doesn't exist down the avenues you've been lead to expect that it would.

First, know that you are absolutely not alone in your pain. We are currently experiencing an epidemic of pain in the United States. According to a study done by The National Institute of Health, 100 million Americans are in pain right now. (1) If our medical system had all the answers, that simply wouldn't be the case.

100 million Americans. That's about a third of our population.

And the statistics only count those who seek treatment for their pain. There may be many more in pain that don't get tabulated in the statistics because, for a myriad of reasons, they aren't going to doctors.

Second, let's get this clear. Chronic pain is a complex condition. It is not curable by one pill or one approach. The fact that your pain hasn't left yet is not your fault.

Is it the fault of our medical system? I don't know, but I do know that we haven't found the answers to chronic pain in pharmaceuticals or medical treatments meant for short-term ailments. For the vast majority of pain sufferers, the present system simply isn't working.

So, how do we understand what this means, how do we find ways to live with the uncertainty, and how do we find an approach that works?First, let's define chronic pain.

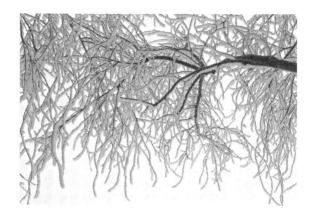

3
DEFINING CHRONIC PAIN

SIMPLY PUT, CHRONIC pain is pain that doesn't end when we think it should. The second half of that definition is, and we don't know how to make it stop.

Here are some quotes from major medical sites on the internet that define chronic pain in slightly fancier words, but say basically the same thing:

Medscape

"Chronic pain syndrome (CPS) is a common problem that presents a major challenge to health-care providers...Some authors suggest that any pain that persists longer than the reasonably expected healing time for the involved tissues should be considered chronic pain." (2)

Medicinenet

"Chronic pain: Pain that persists or progresses over a long period of time...and is often resistant to medical treatments." (3)

NIH Medline Plus

"Chronic pain is often defined as any pain lasting more than 12 weeks...Whatever the treatment plan, it is important to remember that chronic pain usually cannot be cured..." (4)

What do these major medical websites have in common regarding chronic pain?

They don't fully understand it, and they don't have a definitive answer to either treating or curing it.

So, if the medical community is flummoxed by chronic pain, what do we, as chronic pain sufferers, do with this information? How do we find out what it is that we're really involved with here?

When we speak of chronic pain, we're mostly

talking about pain that won't go away over time. That seems simple enough to understand.

Yet we usually seem to think that chronic pain should respond to the same kinds of treatments that we use for short-term pain and, so far, this approach isn't working out all that well for a lot of us. Some of us may be able to put our pain at something of a distance through pharmaceuticals, but we are not actually healing whatever is causing the pain. Living on pharmaceuticals does not seem like much of a cure to me.

So, let's look at why chronic pain and short-term pain don't belong in the same category.

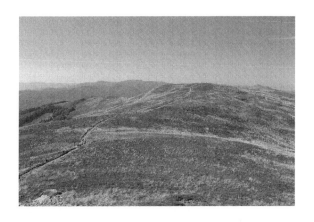

4
HOW CRONIC PAIN IS DIFFERENT
FROM SHORT-TERM PAIN

PAIN IS SOMEWHAT difficult to talk about because, in the English language anyway, we use the one word "pain" for a whole assortment of emotional and physical discomforts.

We have the pain that goes with heartache, and the pain of a stubbed toe. We have pain that stabs and pain that is dull and achey.

We have pain that we are fine with because we know it is necessary, such as the sharp jab from a shot of penicillin for treating an infection. We have pain that lasts a few seconds, and pain that lasts for years.

We have pain that is directly related to an obvious moment when we got hurt, and we have pain that grows slowly over time due to an illness or loss of vitality. And, we have pain that arrives with no known cause at all.

All of these we refer to as "pain".

What we call chronic pain seems to be in its own category. It is dissimilar to short-lived pain in the way it is experienced, felt, generated, and healed. It is altogether a different beast.

In my experience, there are a number of important ways that chronic pain differs from short-term pain. These differences include, but are not limited to, the following:

- While short-term pain can almost always be directly related to a specific injury or illness, chronic pain may lose its relationship to a specific cause over time, or the physical cause may never have been apparent.

- Short-term pain diminishes in intensity and disappears over time, while chronic pain may remain as acute as ever, or may even increase.

- Short-term pain subsides in a fairly predictable pattern, while chronic pain is unpredictable, with spikes and plateaus.

- Short-term pain responds well to rest and treatment; chronic pain responds minimally or not at all.

- Short-term pain usually emanates from the area that is physically impaired; chronic pain may move around the body, seemingly randomly.

- The emotional repercussions of short-term physical pain are also usually short-lived, while chronic pain can have severe and long-term emotional repercussions such as PTSD, hopelessness, depression and suicidal tendencies.

- Most often, short-term pain does not demand that you radically change your lifestyle to get through the ordeal, while chronic pain often requires extensive lifestyle changes.

- Short-term pains are easily understood by others, since most of us have experienced illness or injury at one time or another in our lives; chronic pain is less easily understood, especially by those who expect all pain to respond to medication and are puzzled and even suspicious of reports of pain that never leaves.

I think it is important to notice these differences so that we can begin to look for alternative approaches taylor-made for chronic pain.

Now that we've established that chronic pain is in its own category, we can probably assume that it requires its own approach to pain management and, ultimately, to healing.

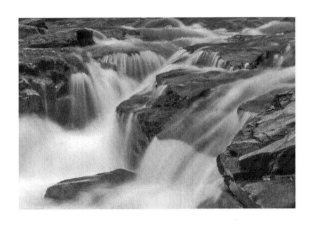

5
SHOULD WE CHANGE OUR
APPROACH TO HEALING?

MANY OF US naturally start our journey with chronic
pain as if it is a short-term situation, of course,
because we don't yet know that it will become
chronic. How could we? There comes a time,
however, when we realize that our pain is not
leaving, and that we may be living with it for an
extended period of time.

It is at this point that we, and our practitioners,
should consider re-assessing our healing strategy
and probably changing gears. Pain clinics and
medical professionals are very aware at this point

that chronic pain is complex and difficult to treat, yet, when pain refuses to leave, the most prevalent approach to pain care offered to the patient is still a long line of prescription drugs.

To me, this is not a viable solution since it really isn't creating health, its creating dependency. We might want to stop putting our energy, financial resources, and time into short-term solutions that aren't working and switch to a new approach.

First, we will have to accept that we may be in this process for some time to come and, therefore, begin to look at possibilities for recovery from new angles and perspectives, tapping into other levels of healing that go beyond purely physical manipulations and chemical substances, and finding approaches that will work for us over the long term.

We will also need to come to grips with how to live with pain day in and day out without losing our minds.

So, how do we know when we've gone from short-term pain to chronic pain?

When Does Pain Become Chronic?

Practitioners vary in what they consider the appropriate timeframe for relabeling pain from just "pain" to "chronic pain".

Some use the 3-month rule. If you've been in pain, either continuous or recurring, for at least 90 days, you've migrated over to the realm of chronic pain.

Some use 6 months as a criterion, and some use whatever they consider "normal" for your condition as the reference point. If you are in pain beyond whatever they would consider reasonable for what ails you, then it is termed "chronic".

In addition to using a timeframe, I've also noticed several more signs that indicate that you may be transitioning from short-term pain to chronic pain:

- Your pain treatments, medications and healing protocols are not significantly changing the type of pain you are in or its intensity. That is, if you stopped all medication today, would you be in nearly the same amount of pain as when you started?

- Your pain levels have risen, rather than diminished, despite treatment or as a result of treatment.

- The pain you are in is puzzling to your practitioner.

- Your pain does not diminish significantly when you rest, or it returns as soon as you are active again.

Once we realize that our pain has become chronic, in what ways do we change our approach to healing?

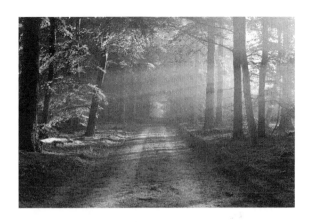

6
ENDING PAIN IS NOT ALWAYS THE BEGINNING

IF PAIN COULD end right away, that would be our preference. But when it doesn't end after weeks and months of therapies, treatments and pills, we need to wonder if putting all our energy into trying to get rid of pain, to kill it, may not be what is called for right now.

Since chronic pain does not respond wholeheartedly to the pain management, treatments, and medications that work for short-term pain, why insist on continuing with the same protocols?

We must first realize that, despite our culture's

fixation on speed for almost everything, there is not going to be a quick fix for the kind of pain we're in. If there was, we would have found it already.

Second, chronic pain is multi-layered, it involves much more than physical discomfort, it also consists of deep emotional components that either come with the pain from the beginning, or develop from the difficulties of living with pain day in and day out.

Third, we need to address the fact that the stresses of living with pain are much higher for those who do not see an end in sight than for those who are clearly on the mend. Lifestyles must be re-designed to accommodate keeping pain to a manageable level, which may require quite severe restrictions on mobility and participation in life.

Painful Entanglements

We've established that short-term pain and long-term pain are different creatures. My feeling is that one of the reasons they are so different and respond to treatment so differently is because long-term pain becomes embedded with both the condition and the emotions that come from living with the condition and living with pain.

Of course, we can reason that pain is not leaving because our condition hasn't healed yet. That makes sense. But what if the condition, which was the cause of our pain in the first place, has become entangled with the ongoing pain in such a way that our continued pain has become part of what is inhibiting the body from healing?

It's as if the condition morphed into something new, multi-leveled, and more complicated. The original condition is now woven into and around the condition of chronic pain such that they are both holding the other in place.

When we make ending pain our primary focus at the beginning of our healing journey, and the pain refuses to go, it may mean we are missing something in our approach.

When we try to get rid of pain through force, instead of soothing, calming, healing, relaxing, and releasing, we are resisting, attacking, and bombarding the pain AND our tired body with chemical substances.

In a strange way, in treating pain as an adversary, we are forcing it to dig in. Somehow, it becomes merged with the original condition, which becomes merged with it, all of which is merged with our physical system. So, trying to treat just one or the other alone doesn't seem to work well.

So the question then becomes, how can we work with chronic pain in a new way, which does not try to kill it but allows it to disentangle itself, so to speak, to begin to move and flow and release the body for full healing?

Since we have been unable to heal our painful condition through purely physical methods, whether traditional or alternative, we want to consider addressing the non-physical aspects of pain as part of our healing path. These would include the emotional and mental components.

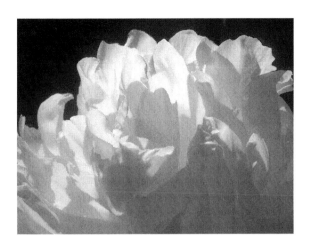

7
NINE APPROACHES TO
MANAGING CHRONIC PAIN

WHEN WE FIRST encounter pain, we usually try to stop it, kill it, silence it, ignore it, hurry it up, get angry with it, or overcome it in some way. What if we tried a very different approach? What would that look like?

We would have to turn our ideas about chronic pain around.

I had a teacher many years ago who told me that if you wanted to change your life, instead of heading in the direction that isn't working and insisting that the circumstances change for you, you stop, turn around and choose a completely different vector.

After years of pushing against the pain in my body, I remembered my teacher's words and took them to heart in regard to the way I was handling my pain. I decided to stop insisting on heading in the direction that wasn't producing the results I wanted.

I decided, instead of trying to end pain as the first step to healing, I would turn toward it and initiate a completely different, more positive relationship with it.

1. ALLOW PAIN TO BE THERE

I know, this feels like the last thing you want to do, but your resistance to the pain you're experiencing in your body may be prolonging its stay. Pain needs to move and it can get stuck in place by the very fact that we refuse to let it be there.

In my experience, and in the experience of many others who have also taken this journey with chronic pain, resisting the pain, hating it, and trying to make it stop actually helps hold it in place.

It does something to kind of freeze a moment in time, as if that will stop the pain, but it seems to just stop it from completing its journey. We get stuck in the moment of pain and, because we refuse to fully feel the pain (understandably, because it hurts!), in a strange way, that moment never ends.

Once you accept that pain is there and you allow it to be there rather than trying to get it to leave, it begins to let up, just a bit. And then a bit more. And then a bit more.

So, the first most important thing you can do to reduce your pain is absolutely counterintuitive. Let your pain be where it is, as it is. Then, make further choices towards healing.

2. GIVE PAIN SPACE

What does it mean to give pain space and why would we want to do that?

When we feel pain we usually pull away from it, physically. This tenses the body and creates more pain. Instead, we're going to go in the opposite direction and give pain more space to relax into.

Right now, try to relax your body around your

pain. Just give the painful areas a little more breathing room and see how that feels.

Try to stop tightening, tensing, contracting and pulling away from the pain. Breathe into the pain and let it relax with you. Imagine more space around the pain in your body.

3. GIVE PAIN TIME

Understand that pain keeps its own timetable. It will leave only when it is ready. It just doesn't respond well to pushing, forcing or demanding it to leave.

Paradoxically, it seems to reduce faster when you give it all the time in the world. Since it hasn't left so far by trying to force it out, it may be more useful to decide to give it, and your body, whatever time it takes to heal fully.

4. LISTEN TO PAIN

Think of chronic pain as someone who has never been listened to, and never fully heard, but has something vital to say. Is it stubborn and recalcitrant, or could it be called dedicated?

What if, instead of trying to torture you, pain was trying to talk to you? What if pain carried a message from you to you and it won't stop until it is delivered?

Consider this: if your pain was a long buried part of you trying to speak to the conscious, everyday, you, what would it be saying?

5. TREAT PAIN GENTLY

Instead of yelling at pain and pushing against it, treat it (and yourself) more gently.

Right now, soften your stance against pain.

In fact, instead of being against pain, imagine that you are, in some way, just being with pain. Being next to pain.

Allow pain its place in your body for the moment.

Is there any way you can soften your stance toward yourself too? Maybe stop blaming yourself for being in pain.

Maybe stop asking yourself to get better faster.

Maybe stop expecting yourself to have all the answers right now, today.

6. LET YOURSELF FEEL

It is important to understand that we are creatures

of physical, mental, emotional and spiritual aspects.

Chronic pain seems to be wound around all of these in some way, which is why I believe that treating it as a purely physical condition isn't working for most people.

We talked about letting yourself feel the physical pain in your body as a starting point. I believe that it is also important to let yourself feel the emotional components of being in pain.

This can be challenging, because the last thing you want to do is feel more pain. You can barely stand the physical pain you're in, so why would you want to feel any emotional pain you might be experiencing too?

Usually we want to ignore them so we can get through the day. When a strong emotion comes up we usually try to stuff it back down again because it just seems like too much for us to handle both kinds of pain, physical and emotional.

The trouble with this method, even though it is highly understandable, it that it just isn't helpful. In my experience, and in the experience of others I have worked with who have also had to live with chronic pain, the emotions of living in pain become intertwined with the physical aspects of living with pain. Not allowing your emotions to be felt may be another way you are keeping pain in place.

Letting emotions move and flow helps your physical pain move on.

I am not saying that all chronic pain is the product of deeply repressed emotions, although I know some people hold that theory to be true.

What I'm saying here is that there are going to be deep emotions that arise from the experience of having your life significantly altered by pain and from having to live in physical discomfort day in and day out.

It's unavoidable. It can be sad, lonely, distressing and maddeningly frustrating. You may feel hopeless, depressed, angry, betrayed, lost, or terrified. Or you could run through all of those in one day.

Pain medications may be numbing your physical pain and that may help you rest and sleep and that can be a good thing, but be careful that you are not also numbing your emotional responses as well.

We're afraid that if we allow ourselves to feel our

deep emotional responses to pain, that we'll wallow in self-pity, or start crying in front of our doctor, or get so angry that we'll do something we regret.

In my experience, however, the uncontrolled expressions of our feelings are not the result of allowing them to be felt, they are the result of suppressing them over time and then they leak or burst out when it's least convenient.

Feelings don't just go away. They congeal.

Find ways to feel your feelings, and to acknowledge them as they arise as much as you can. Help your feelings not become calcified energy that imprisons pain within them.

Here are some suggestions for ways to honor and express the emotional side of living with chronic pain.

7. KEEP A JOURNAL

Talk to yourself about the emotions you are feeling by writing them down in a journal. You can even draw them if you want, or paste in pictures from magazines that illustrate what you're feeling.

Cry over them, wrestle with them, but find a way

to let them be felt and then to move on, even if you have to do this as a daily exercise.

It is so much healthier than numbing yourself out, refusing to allow yourself to feel, or waiting until they burst out of you like the steam from a tea kettle.

8. FIND SOMEONE TO TALK TO

Find someone you can express your feelings to that will not feel sorry for you, try to fix you, or feel like you are dumping on them.

This takes a special kind of person who is able to listen without taking anything on, or taking it personally.

If you don't have someone like that in your life, and, I admit they are rare, consider paying for a therapy session now and then if you can afford it.

If that's not possible, another option is to tell your story to Nature. I know it may sound odd, but talking to the ocean, a tree, the breeze, or the moon is way better than keeping things bottled up. I find that at least in Nature, there is a real feeling of a presence there, listening in some inexplicable way. If you haven't tried this before, give it a go. You may be pleasantly surprised at how much better you feel.

9. SCHEDULE CHECK-INS
WITH YOURSELF

Consider choosing a set time at least once a week when you have an appointment to check in with your emotional life.

Use this time to check in with yourself about what you're going through. You don't even have to know what label to put on your emotions, just feel what you are feeling. Let them move so you don't keep them locked into place with your physical pain, or your pain locked in place with unexpressed emotional goo.

Listen to evocative music, do some creative dance movement, make doodle art or other kinds of crafts, or take a walk in nature.

However you choose to do this, it is so important that you feel your feelings in order to help your pain move on. Don't let your unfelt emotions help keep pain in place.

SUMMARY

1. ALLOW PAIN TO BE THERE

2. GIVE PAIN SPACE

3. GIVE PAIN TIME

4. LISTEN TO PAIN

5. TREAT PAIN GENTLY

6. LET YOURSELF FEEL

7. KEEP A JOURNAL

8. FIND SOMEONE TO TALK TO

9. SCHEDULE CHECK-INS WITH YOURSELF

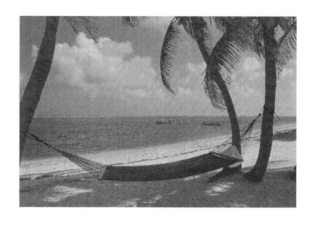

8
TWELVE MORE WAYS TO MAKE
LIFE EASIER TODAY

WE MAY NOT be able to end pain overnight, but we can find ways to make life easier for ourselves during the time we are living with pain. Here are some practical steps that helped me. Most of them you can make use of today to create more ease and relief in your life right now.

1. BE WILLING TO SLOW WAY, WAY DOWN

You have to be willing to not do a whole lot.

If you're a go-getter, an active person, a parent, a manager, an athlete or anyone else used to moving fast, being a leader, and getting a lot done, this is really hard. You have to be fairly ruthless with yourself. You have to stop yourself from taking care of everything, making sure everyone is alright, organizing stuff and being a Type A. You just do.

For right now, you're going to need to let go of some of your control.

Well, a lot of your control.

You have to let things be done less well than the way you would like them to be done. You have to let other people do things for you, even if they do them badly in your opinion. That just has to be okay for now. Doing things perfectly isn't perfect right now. What's perfect for you is letting go of taking care of everything you used to take care of.

I know how hard this is, but the longer you try to be the person you were when you didn't have pain, and the longer you refuse to give yourself a break, chances are, the longer your pain will be with you.

2. REDUCE STRESS

First and foremost, stress heightens pain. There is no getting around it. Prolonged stress is bad for the body. In fact, many physicians now believe that stress is the primary factor in creating disease in the body to begin with. Whether your pain is from illness or injury, stress is not doing you any good.

You're going to have challenges when you're in pain because your body is simply not able to do what it used to do. You may not be able to work as many hours, or at all. This is going to create financial worries, as well as worries about missing work and not being able to keep up with those demands, and possibly losing opportunities for advancement. You may feel you have to hide your pain at work, which is stressful in itself.

In addition, your medical insurance may not cover all your expenses. You've got doctor's visits, tests, procedures and medical decisions to worry about, while still trying to maintain some kind of normalcy in your relationships with your family and friends.

How do you do this without getting totally stressed out and raising your pain levels?

It's not easy, I know. The first thing I want to tell you from my own experience is that stressing out about it is not going to make things easier or better for you. Give as many stressful problems and tasks away as you can for the time being. Allow other people to handle things for you as much as possible. This is so important when you're in pain, that I reiterate it several times in this book. Please make life easier for yourself right now.

We worry that things won't get done unless we do them, and we may be right. But at this point, the most important thing you can do for yourself is allow your body to find a way to rest, heal, and regenerate.

We often don't realize how much choice we actually have around how much we stress about things. But worrying and stressing is a response to our situation that we do have control over. We can choose to respond differently.

Once you understand that stress actually creates more pain, you can come to an agreement within yourself that you simply can't afford to let yourself get stressed. Stressing will only prolong the time it takes you to heal, which will lead to even more stress and more worries. It's a vicious circle.

Most of the suggestions in this book will help reduce stress.

3. SIMPLIFY (BECOME VERY ZEN)

Since anxiety put my pain levels through the roof, and I'd realized that I needed to de-stress as much as possible, I decided to adopt a lifestyle that was very, very simple and very, very calm.

I simplified my life as much as I could, cutting back on any and all things that absolutely didn't need doing right then. I dropped a lot out of my life.

This means that I had to change my priorities hugely. I had to re-categorize almost everything so that all the things that weren't absolutely necessary pretty much fell off my to-do list entirely. When I was in acute pain, what remained on the list (after personal hygiene and eating) was only one or two absolute necessities in a day.

I'm not kidding. One or two absolute necessities. Going to one appointment. Making one important phone call that required organization and brain power. Resting the remainder of the day.

To someone who is not in pain, this sounds

ludicrous. How can you only do one or two things in a day? If you are in pain, however, that may be all you can do without spiking pain levels. If that.

From my limited exposure to Zen Buddhist art and Zen Buddhist principles which, to me, seem to exemplify calm simplicity, I called this becoming very "Zen". I didn't find that I could meditate very well in pain, but I could use the principles of minimalism that went with the Zen lifestyle.

I deliberately started moving more slowly and calmly, and breathing more slowly and calmly. Try it. I think you'll find that if you do this, within one day, you will feel better.

(If you think you absolutely can't reduce your list of what must get done in a day, even when you're in extreme pain, see 6. Ask for Help Often)

4. DECIDE TO STOP WORRYING

I made a conscious choice to stop worrying about what happened, what might happen, and what could happen. I decided that my primary occupation was to get better. That was what I was about. I no longer had the luxury of stress and worry. I just couldn't afford it, physically.

I focused on calm breathing, not letting things get to me, and telling myself over and over that right now, everything was okay, and that everything was going to work out, one way or another.

I consciously put my worries aside (realizing that worrying wasn't going to change anything anyway), and made some careful choices about the few things I was going to be able to do in a given day. I stuck to only those few things (and many times had to say no to a lot of things I used to be able to do).

I made this a way of life. In a way, it was almost like a religious vow. It was a commitment to myself that I took very seriously and honored as I would honor any business, spiritual, or relationship commitment.

As I did this, things started to change. My pain levels became less acute, my body relaxed more, and I felt better in general, even while I was still experiencing pain. I slept a little more soundly and a little bit longer, so I began to feel somewhat better during the day.

This is not an easy thing to do, I admit. But it is

really important if you are going to get your pain levels under control. I suggest that you make this kind of commitment to yourself and make healing your absolute top priority. And, although it sounds like a priority is something you do, as we've said before, healing is often a whole lot of not-doing.

5. TAKE MANY SMALL RESTS

It's hard to get a good night's sleep when you're in pain. You toss and turn, adjust the pillows, get up and make tea, turn on the computer or the TV, go back to bed, and start the whole thing over again.

Once we've done that all night, for some reason we seem to think we're supposed to get up in the morning and act like it's a normal day. It isn't. You're exhausted. Whenever you can, during the day, make time for as many small rest periods as possible. If you're still working full time while in pain, then you will have to be creative about it.

Resting does not just mean stopping what you're doing. It means slowing yourself down on the inside too. It means taking a few slow, deep breaths, closing your eyes and not thinking about anything in particular. It means letting yourself feel your body, and be with your body, even in and with the pain.

I know that doesn't sound very restful, but most of the time we are consciously or unconsciously resisting the pain we're in and that takes more energy than you realize. It is actually more productive to give yourself a few moments to feel how you feel, acknowledge it to yourself, breathe, relax around the pain, relax with the pain and let it be, than it is to expend energy trying to override the pain and carry on without these rest periods.

So, give yourself a break. Rest often throughout the day. If you are already confined to bed, make sure that your time there is actually as relaxed and calm as it can be. Remember to stop on the inside too.

6. ASK FOR HELP OFTEN

Most of us are terrible about asking for help from others, especially strangers. If you're in pain, you're going to need to get over it. If there is something that will cause a spike in pain levels either immediately or later and someone else can easily do it, ask for help.

Ask for help often.

Ask for help with household chores, filling out forms, getting to the doctor, cooking dinner, answering emails, and making appointments. Don't think that the things you need help with are too small to bother people with.

If it fatigues you to do them, if it will increase the amount of pain you are in now or later, ask people around you to do these things for you.

Because using my arms and hands is painful with my condition, I've had to get used to asking others to open doors, pull out chairs, open jars, and carry grocery bags or plates of food.

I never used to have to ask for help for hardly anything, so this level of vulnerability was foreign to me and I was really uncomfortable with it at first. What I found out, however, was that most people are perfectly happy to help if you just ask politely.

Most of us have learned to suffer in silence and carry on despite any discomfort we're in, as if that's somehow heroic. It really isn't. You just can't do that anymore and heal your body.

Of course, be aware of not over-burdening others by asking the same few people to do everything. See if you can spread it around a bit. There may also be nonprofit agencies in your area that have services for people in pain, or you might reach out to people in your church or other community organizations.

Remember, most of us err on the side of trying to do it all ourselves, and this is really not the time for that.

7. LET GO OF YOUR SCHEDULE FOR HEALING

It is the nature of chronic pain to stick around, whether it is penciled in for next Tuesday or not.

It requires a certain kind of emotional balance to neither insist that pain leave (and be constantly disappointed) nor give up hope altogether. The best way I have found to handle the fact that pain isn't leaving is to let go of my scheduled healing date.

As much as we want it to end right now, our ideas of how long pain should stick around don't seem to be of much concern to pain. Pain has its own purpose, its own timeframe, and its own requirements for what needs to happen before it will leave. We only end up discouraged if we keep noticing how long we've already been in pain, and fretting about how long it will be before we're out of pain.

This doesn't mean we give up hope, not at all. But I've found that a better way to be with pain, and one which, paradoxically seems to ease it, is to resolve to give it the time it needs.

This seems like an acquiescence to pain that we certainly don't want to make, I know. But pain is here anyway, and fretting about when it will end creates a kind of tension and stress that is not conducive to the relaxation and calm we need to heal. It has a lot to do with allowing what is already happening to be happening, rather than insisting that it be different.

Make a habit of writing in any progress you see from week to week in your schedule book instead.

8. TAKE MINI HEALING VACATIONS

Find ways to give yourself little mini vacations either physically or in your mind. If you can get out to a beautiful park or other natural area, or you can treat yourself to a very gentle massage, or even just a long soak in the bathtub with candles and bubble bath, give yourself little pleasant vacations like these. Yes, of course, pain is going to come along for the ride, but that's okay for now. Imagine your pain is also enjoying the scenery or the soak.

If you can't do anything physical, take a mini vacation in your mind. Put on some nice music, find some pictures of beautiful scenery or have someone print some off the internet for you. Use these as aides in imagining that you are somewhere very relaxing.

You can even imagine that pain is in the beach chair next to you, just taking a breather.

9. FIND A TRIBE

Do the best you can to find a community of people who are facing similar challenges as you, either through a local meet-up group, a charity, or online. It just helps tremendously to know that others are out there also looking for ways to live with and live through this time with pain without losing their ability to continue to experience some of the positive aspects of life.

The benefits of finding a tribe are more important than you might first think. I really didn't feel well enough to seek others out when I was first injured, and it was a number of years into my pain journey before I connected with other people who were also experiencing chronic pain.

I was surprised by the level of relief I discovered in just knowing a few other people who really understood the emotional and psychological challenges of pain, as well as the physical aspects.

Besides the sense of finally being truly seen and understood, a tribe offers you the possibility that someone will have a suggestion that helps you out a great deal. You may also have some sound advice or a little piece of wisdom to offer someone else.

Having something to contribute to others when you are shut out of many of life's normal pleasures and interactions can help relieve the isolation that often accompanies living with pain.

I think the most important aspects of having a tribe is knowing there are others who understand, who know what this path is like, who don't need you to heal faster or wonder if you aren't trying hard enough; that there is a place (even if it's only in cyberspace) to meet regularly; and that you are not alone.

If there is no existing group that you can find, consider starting one.

10. UNDERSTAND YOUR PAIN-O-METER

I suggest that you get in touch with your inner Pain-O-Meter. Basically, this means becoming familiar in the most intimate terms with what actions, feelings, and stressors trigger or spike your pain. When you are intimate with your pain triggers you can do a better job of regulating what you say yes and no to in any given day, and when to best schedule any activities you plan on doing.

So, the Pain-O-Meter is my way of describing the awareness you have of your pain levels over time.

The most useful way I've found to monitor my pain levels is to keep a pain diary. Sounds pretty dismal, I know, but it can be a very helpful tool.

A pain diary does not have to be anything

elaborate, just a way to note down the time, type of pain, and level of pain you experience over the course of a day and continue this for at least a week. This is most useful if you also note your current mood, what you're doing, and any stressors present at the moment.

This way you can corollate what you are feeling and doing, the time of day, when you rest and when you're active, with how these affect your pain levels.

So, for example, you may find out, as I did, that, contrary to what I would have assumed to be true, mornings were a terrible time to try to plan appointments. I was not more rested and refreshed in the morning.

I usually arose feeling like I'd been hit by a train, exhausted from tossing and turning and trying to get comfortable enough to catnap until my pain levels rose and woke me again. Arising after that experience, doing my personal hygiene routine and then having to be somewhere at a particular time usually created significant increases in pain levels.

Tracking your pain makes you aware of any recurring patterns that you might otherwise not have noticed. You can make a little more sense of your pain rhythms during the day. Noticing them allows you to plan around them. If you're aware of what sets off your Pain-O-Meter, you can plan to rest more often when the inner gauge most often registers "high" pain levels, and plan to take care of necessary tasks when your inner gauge most often seems to read "low".

You can download a free PDF which you can use as a basis for your pain monitor from my website here.

11. MAKE FRIENDS WITH PAIN

I know this is counterintuitive, but it is really helpful to make friends with the pain in your body as best you can. It's not something we do naturally, and it seems almost like a self-betrayal at first. Why should I befriend the thing that is causing me so much distress?

Trying to fight with pain only makes things worse. It causes you to tense up more, it's frustrating, it usually doesn't work, and it's emotionally and physically exhausting.

Accept that pain is in your body right now. That seems obvious, but most of us skip right over that step. Just accept that there is pain, without trying to force it away from you. It doesn't feel good, I understand, but pushing against it will not make it feel better. Quite the opposite.

Okay, so I'm accepting my pain, you say, with your arms crossed. So now, send some friendly energy to your pain. Send it a sense of goodwill. This too seems absolutely like the last thing you want to do. Why would want to give pain anything at all?

Try this right now. Take a deep breath, let it out with a sigh, and for several moments, stop fighting your pain and see it as a friendly force. Imagine that your pain has a positive purpose. It really isn't trying to torture you. It is trying to heal you and move on. Release any tightness or gripping around the painful area. Imagine pain flowing onward to wherever it wants to go. What happens?

Know that pain is in your body for a reason. You may not fully understand it right now, but it has a purpose for being there. Use its fluctuations as a signal to tell you when you've gone too far physically for one day. Listen to it. Use pain to inform you of the kind of emotions and thoughts that trigger it.

Tune into your Pain-O-Meter not as an evil tyrant, but as a useful gauge that is helping you understand what activities, what attitudes, and what approaches are helping you heal, and which ones you should avoid.

12. HOLD YOURSELF BLAMELESS

Finally, but not least importantly, give yourself a lot of emotional leeway. You are doing the best you can to deal with the daily challenges of living in and with pain and it's not easy. You are healing as fast as you can, even if that seems like a snail's pace to you. If you could do anything better than you are now, you would.

Give yourself a pat on the back (metaphorically if that's painful) just for getting through another day. You are walking a very difficult path. You may not understand the reason for this path, but, one way or another, you are on it.

Be as kind to yourself as you would be to a small child who is hurting. Be gentle, be reasonably positive, let yourself have a good cry when you need it, then brush the dirt off your knees and lift your eyes off the ground.

Yes, sometimes we wish we could have a kind parent or friend do this for us, but often we have to do this for ourselves. And we can. And when we find others to talk to, to cry with, to share with, we offer them the kindnesses we also need for ourselves.

SUMMARY

1. BE WILLING TO SLOW WAY, WAY DOWN

2. REDUCE STRESS

3. SIMPLIFY (BECOME VERY ZEN)

4. DECIDE TO STOP WORRYING

5. TAKE MANY SMALL RESTS

6. ASK FOR HELP OFTEN

7. LET GO OF YOUR SCHEDULE FOR HEALING

8. TAKE MINI HEALING VACATIONS

9. FIND A TRIBE

10. UNDERSTAND YOUR PAIN-O-METER

11. MAKE FRIENDS WITH PAIN

12. HOLD YOURSELF BLAMELESS

NOTES

(1) National Institutes of Health, Final Report, Pathways to Prevention Workshop: The Role of Opioids in the Treatment of Chronic Pain, Setember 29-30, 2014, Executive Summary, p. 1

(2) Singh, Manish K, MD, Chronic Pain Syndrome, Medscape website:

www.medicinenet.com/chronic_pain/symptoms.htm

(3) Shiel, William C. Jr., MD, FACP, FACR, Chronic Pain Early Symptoms & Signs, MedicineNet.com:

www.medicinenet.com/chronic_pain/symptoms.htm

(4) NIH MedlinePlus, Chronic Pain: Symptoms, Diagnosis & Treatment, NIH Medline Plus website:

www.nlm.nih.gov/medlineplus/magazine/issues/spring1 1/articles/spring11pg5-6.html

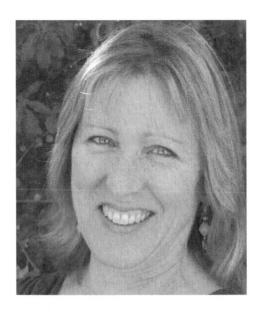

ABOUT THE AUTHOR

A native of Connecticut, Sarah Anne Shockley is a multiple award winning producer and director of educational films, including *Dancing From the Inside Out*, a highly acclaimed documentary on disabled dance. She has traveled extensively for business and pleasure. Her first book, *Traveling Incognito*, a guidebook for international travelers, won a Critic's Choice Award (San Francisco Review of Books). She holds an MBA in International Marketing and has worked in high-tech management, as a corporate trainer, and teaching undergraduate and graduate business administration. As the result of a work related injury in the Fall of 2007, Sarah contracted Thoracic Outlet Syndrome (TOS) and has lived with debilitating nerve pain since then. She currently resides in the San Francisco Bay Area with her son.

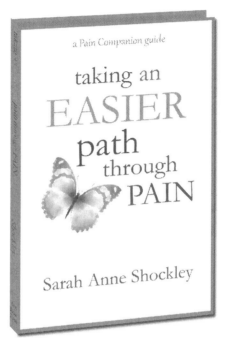

a Pain Companion guide

taking an

EASIER

path
through
PAIN

Sarah Anne Shockley

Taking An Easier Path Through Pain discusses 10 prevalent ways that chronic pain affects daily life and offers useful suggestions for mitigating their impact.

PLEASE VISIT www.ThePainCompanion.com to register for your FREE COPY of *Taking An Easier Path Through Pain.*

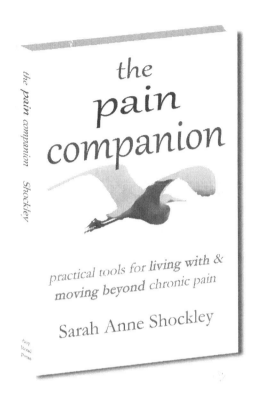

The Pain Companion: Practical Tools for Living With and Moving Beyond Chronic Pain, Paperback, 2016, 176 pages, $14.95

The Pain Companion is based on the author's 8 years of managing debilitating nerve pain. It contains a wealth of insights and wisdom to help mitigate the impact that living with chronic pain has on emotional well being, self-image and relationships. It includes 33 specific ways to mitigate pain's emotional, mental, and physical stresses, and 11 easy meditative exercises to establish communication with pain in the body and enlist pain as an ally in healing.

PLEASE VISIT www.ThePainCompanion.com for sample chapters from *The Pain Companion.*

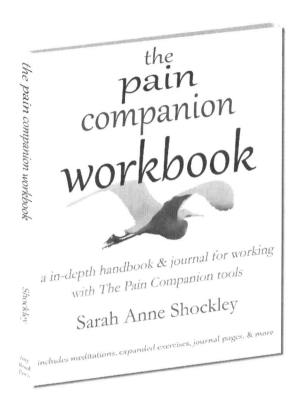

The Pain Companion Workbook: 16 Meditative Exercises for Relieving Chronic Pain, Paperback, 2016

The Pain Companion Workbook expands and broadens the scope of each of the meditative exercises from The Pain Companion for readers who wish to explore their relationship to pain, to life, and to themselves on a deeper level. Includes space for fully responding to the exercises, journaling prompts, a pain diary, and 5 additional exercises not included in *The Pain Companion.*

Made in the USA
San Bernardino, CA
05 September 2016